THE QUICK VEDIC GUIDE

TO

HEALING YOUR EMOTIONS

MIRA OM

Why is emotional healing so critical to our wellbeing? Emotions affect the health of the mind, body, and soul. In the Ayurvedic model, our mind and emotions reside in the head and heart in the forms of contentment, clarity, and love. These are governed by the three doshas—*vata* (like the wind), *pitta* (like the fire), and *kapha* (like the water). And in the gut, our third level of emotions stored are of fire or will power, and a little lower, feeling grounded, wanted, or secure. We are all on a soul journey, and you may be conscious or unconscious of this aspect. However, nobody can escape their emotions, whether they are spiritually inclined or not. A big part of the soul journey involves the emotions: healing them, or transcending their challenging aspects. The soul is essentially shaped by the emotional repercussions of its life journey and the challenges we succeed in facing. The achievement of emotional growth as an outcome is the prize.

On the brighter side of the matrix are the gifts we have to offer to the world with our talents, skills, and dreams. While we are comfortable with our gifts and eager to embrace opportunities, it is much more trying to get over challenges, especially those that reside deep within the psyche. This may manifest itself as a tendency to be hypercritical or quick to anger, to withdraw and give up, or an inability to let go. It is easier to sabotage ourselves with our negative emotions than with our mental or physical shortcomings.

In the modern world, the most popularly practiced methods of altering or balancing the emotions are positive affirmations, meditation, psychotherapy, and a doctor's prescription. However, Ayurveda has a much bigger toolbox. In addition to whatever works for you, incorporating a little of everything — all the sensory and organic therapies — will speed up and ease your goal towards emotional balance.

While Western medicine thinks the mind can only be healed through the mind, Ayurveda knows that the mind can be healed through the senses and the body as well. Using these therapies will not tax your willpower because most of the therapies are physically implemented. There are three major doshas, and a combination of the three creates a total of seven types; however, one primary set of your emotions will be in imbalance to begin with. Don't be afraid to balance; you will not lose any core emotional strength. You will only gain beauty, wisdom, and fortitude. To find your dosha, go to https://miraom.com/free-stuff/.

Ayurveda emerged from the Vedas, an ancient body of wisdom revealed by spiritual *rishis* or seers in India. Even though it is a very ancient knowledge system, it works (surprisingly so, to many living in Western nations) efficiently and logically. Ayurveda offers a practical and pragmatic approach to life and makes tangible the ability to step into a higher, more glorious version of ourselves.

Try it; it works!
Namaste…

Mira Om

www.miraom.com

© Mira 2019

Contents

Vata Emotional Therapy
- *Pacifies the Wind*

Balanced Vata:	Joyful, enthusiastic, and versatile
Imbalanced:	Nervous, scattered, fearful, anxious, and worried
Self-actualized:	Life-enriching joy, teacher, healer, and artist
Key to balance:	Slowdown, structure, and grounding.

The scattering vata energies need to be bounded and grounded. Imbalanced vata emotions take a toll on the mind and *basti* (gut) marma seat, which is the seat of security, or fear when imbalanced, in the lower pelvic area. Each of these therapies work towards getting you centered and strengthened.

Emotion to Cultivate

Faith and surrendering to the Divine, decreasing dependency on the outside world.

Body Parts Susceptible to Imbalanced Emotions

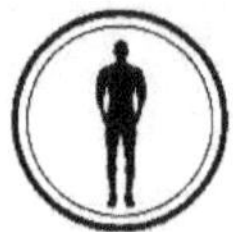

Colon, bones, and nervous system; dryness issues.

Sound

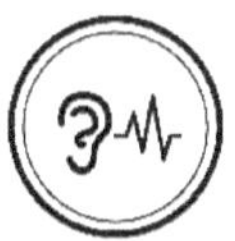

RAM (fiery solar-plex chakra), VAM (watery sacral chakra), and LAM (grounding root chakra).

Color

Warm and moistening colors: gold, red, orange, and yellow; or calming: with limited white.

Aroma/ Essential oil

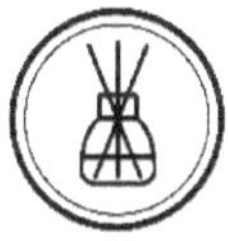

Lavender (soothes nerves), sandalwood (grounding and calms the mind), lotus (calms the heart and mind, and supports deep sleep,

builds *ojas)*, frankincense (spiritually awakening and increases faith), cinnamon (stimulates circulation and warming), basil (clears
stagnating downward force), and camphor
(cleansing and stimulating), cedar (sweet and
warm), myrrh (healing, particularly bones
and nerves, spiritual awakening).

It can be added to slightly warm sesame oil
and apply to crown chakra, third-eye chakra,
and belly.

Gemstones

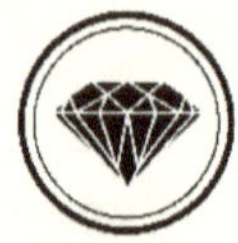

Ruby (concentration and willpower), pearl
(calming and protective), red coral (improves
blood and energy), yellow sapphire (*ojas /*
nourishing), bloodstone (creativity, inspiring,
and harmonizing).

Better results attained with energy healing, such as reiki. Specifically with throat/navel chakra and *basti* (water/root) chakra.

Pranayama

Brahmari (grounding and warming). Alternative nostril breathing (balances nervous system).

Asana

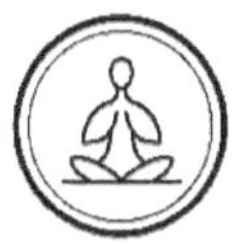

Slow and steady sun salutation, intoxicating bliss pose, or *ananda madirasana.*

Meditation

Avoid excessive meditation; visualization or mantra meditation is more effective, or *yoga nidra*.

Environment

Warm, moist, secure, and safe. Avoid over-stimulation and multi-tasking. Create a peaceful and comfortable space.

Pitta Emotional Therapy
- Cools the Fire

Balanced:	Ambitious, achievers, and active
Imbalanced:	Workaholic, driven, angry, irritable, and jealous
Self-actualized:	Gentle inner light, connecting to the truth; leader, and pioneer
Key to balance:	Leisure and cooling.

The hot-driven pitta energies need to be cooled and reduced. Imbalanced pitta emotions take a toll on the liver and *hrdiya* (heart) marma in the chest, which is the seat of compassion, or coldness when imbalanced. Each of these therapies work towards getting you calmer and softened.

Emotion to cultivate

Forgiveness, compassion, artistic creativity, and surrendering anger.

Body parts susceptible to imbalanced emotions

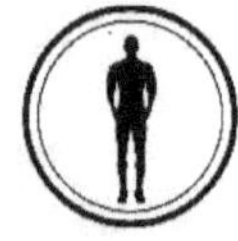

Blood, small intestine, and liver; inflammation issues.

Sound

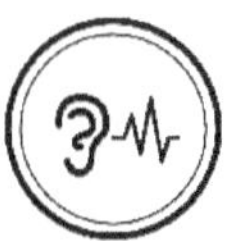

YAM (airy heart chakra) and VAM (watery sacral chakra).

Color

Cooling colors: White, green, blue, and pastels.

Aroma/ Essential oil

Sandalwood (cooling and grounding), vetiver (cools heat from the head), lemongrass (cooling, soothes fevers), lotus (calms heart and mind, and supports deep sleep, builds *ojas*), flower essences — rose (cooling and opens heart chakra), lavender (calming and increases contentment), lily (calms heart), saffron (strengthens love and cleanses blood), gardenia (cleans blood and infections) honeysuckle (cools brain and blood), and iris (cleans, and calms jealousy, anger, and envy).

It can be added to slightly warm ghee, or coconut oil, apply to head and heart chakra.

Gemstones

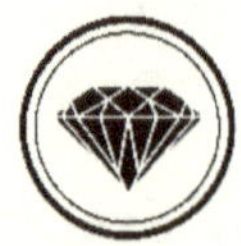

Jade (calming), pearl (calming and protective), amethyst (healing visions, soothes fire), emerald (calms mental agitation and improves intelligence); better results attained with energy medicine- reiki, and especially with the heart and throat/navel chakra.

Pranayama

Sheetali (cooling).

Asana

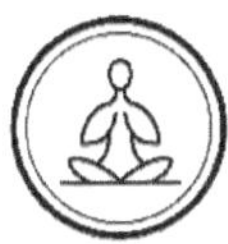

Lunar salutations (cooling) and *moon-pose* with *ujjayi* pranayama.

Meditation

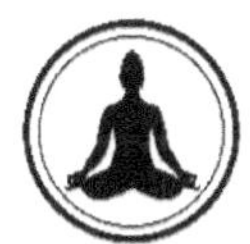

Meditation: Visualization on the moon, water bodies, and meditating on the breath.

Environment

Fun, cheerful, and happy. Meet friends and be creative. Avoid aggression and burnouts.

Kapha Emotional Therapy
- Lightens the Heavy Water

Balanced:	Enduring, patient, and loving
Imbalanced:	Stubborn, depression, lethargy, over-attached, and greed
Self-actualized:	Humanitarian and compassionate nurturer
Key to balance:	Active, lightness, and giving.

The cloistering kapha energies need to be aerated, released, and lightened. Imbalanced kapha emotions take a toll on the heaviness of the body and the *Adipati* (crown) marma on the top of the head, which is the seat of contentment, or confusion when imbalanced. Each of these therapies work towards making you lighter and free.

Emotion to cultivate

Detachment and letting go.

Body parts susceptible to imbalanced emotions

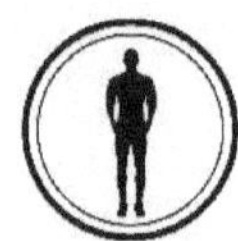

Chest and stomach; watery issues.

Sound

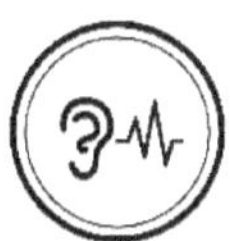

RAM (fiery solar-plex chakra), HAM (space element- throat chakra), and YAM (airy heart chakra)

Color

Vibrant and warm colors — red, orange, yellow, and gold.

Aroma/ Essential oil

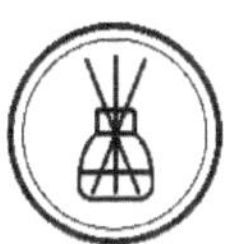

Camphor (opens senses and lungs, and enhances perception and meditation), cinnamon (stimulates circulation), *heena* (promotes clarity and perception), cloves (awakens senses and is a decongestant), musk (fiery and stimulating or *rajasic*), sage (spiritually balancing and uplifting), thyme (strengthens lungs and immunity), cedar (clears edema and strengthens lungs), frankincense (cleanser and removes negative psychic thoughts*), and myrrh (spiritual awakening), patchouli (stimulating and gives joy).

It can be added to slightly warm mix of mustard and sesame oil, or almond oil, and apply to crown chakra, chest, and sinus.

Gemstones

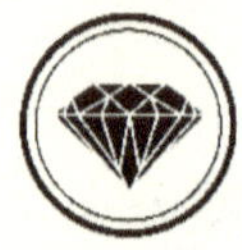

Ruby (fire and willpower), Opal (intensity and passion), blue sapphire (detaching and reducing); better results occur when combined

with energy medicine- reiki, especially at na-
vel/ throat and crown chakra.

Pranayama

Bhastrika (invigorating)

Asana

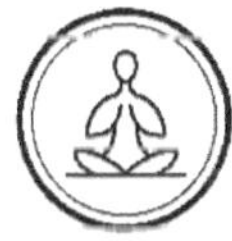

Vigorous poses and back bending like snake
pose (unblocks emotions), and twisting poses
like half-spinal twist (stimulates adrenaline).

Meditation

Active meditation (chanting /vibratory) or
walking meditation.

Environment

Mentally stimulating and austere, dry environment. Challenging the mind with learning and talking. Avoid cluttering, dull, cold, and damp.

Research/Suggested Reading:

1. *Asana Pranayama Mudra Bandha* by Swami Satyananda Saraswati

2. *Edgar Cayce readings on Gemstones at <u>edgarcayce.org</u>

3. *Marma Therapy: The Healing Power of Ayurvedic Vital Point Massage* by Dr. Ernst Schrott (Author), Dr. J. Ramanuja Raju (Author), Stefan Schrott (Author), Marek Lorys (Translator)

4. *The Ayurveda Encyclopedia: Natural Secrets to Healing, Prevention, & Longevity* by Swami Sadashiva Tirtha